Introduction

Meditation: It's as simple as breathing and as difficult as relaxing your thoughts.

Everyone's year in meditation will look and feel a little different, but mine started after more than a decade of yoga, which connects movement and breathing and was originally designed to help people get more comfortable in their bodies, so they could sit in quiet meditation for hours at a time. As a moving form of meditation, I found yoga to be beautiful, inspiring, calming, grounding. I was ready for the next step.

While I know that meditation can be beneficial and perhaps even life-altering, I really, really struggled with it. I could sit still for about two or three minutes, but then my mind would get busy, then my body would want to fidget. It's a familiar story.

So I dedicated myself to trying different forms of meditation, different styles, different times of day as a way of calming my mind, relaxing my body, opening up and tuning in. Likewise, I recognized that yoga is a true pastime and passion for millions of Americans who are enraptured with down dog these days. That's not necessarily the case with meditation.

Meditation can be pretty challenging – whether it's the sitting still part, the various twinges, aches and pains in the body, or our busy, busy minds that are far more comfortable doing 14 things than just one – we struggle to commit to meditation, even though we know it's good for us. And it is very, very good for us.

Meditation is a health and wellness tradition with longevity and an impressive track record. For starters, it's free, and it's something you can do anytime, anywhere (even in traffic, even in a big meeting, even in an argument). It helps reduce stress, increase lung capacity, promote better sleep, boost memory, build immunity, promote detachment, calm, joy and compassion. In recent studies, meditation has even been shown to increase the density of gray matter in parts of the brain associated with memory, stress, regulation of emotions and more. And the list goes on. Meditation can help with everything from relationships to the office, from self-esteem to focus, from weight loss to energy.

With all of that in mind, following are 52 different meditation techniques you can employ to increase empathy and decrease fatigue, to find balance and let go of judgment each week. You can practice them in order, or jump around. If you find something you absolutely love, you're welcome to stick with it for more than a week (and vice versa, although sometimes we need to give the things that challenge us a second chance). If something isn't working, try a little patience and a little softness, but if it still isn't working, try something new! There are a million ways to meditate. As long as you are slowing down and breathing, that's what really matters.

In a year, you will have a consistent meditation practice and more benefits than you could wish for with any New Year's resolution. Breathe in, breathe out, breathe in, breath out, and enjoy.

Getting Started

While meditation is free and adaptable, if you can make it part of your daily routine, you're far more likely to stick with it for the long run. The following tips can help you get – and stay – going:

- Determine when you will meditate each day. Many meditation teachers recommend first thing in the morning before the rat race begins – all you have to do is rise, find a comfortable place to sit and breathe. If you're more of a night owl, nighttime can also work well, giving you the chance to wind down and relax before bed. Either way, try to pick a time and make a date with yourself.

- Find a consistent place to meditate. While your bed might seem ideal, it's actually not – it's too easy to fall asleep there. If you can find a small space in a room where you can sit on the floor and breathe easy, that's ideal; you might want to have some pillows or blankets nearby to sit on. You can also sit in a chair if that just works better for you – just make sure your feet rest comfortably on the floor.

- Prop yourself up. Unless your hips are very flexible and you have zero back pain, sitting flat on the floor for several minutes at a time can be uncomfortable. Sit on the edge of a blanket (or towels or a firm pillow) or even up against a wall. You can also place pillows under your knees for support. The less you have to worry about your posture, the more you can focus on breathing.

- Get personal: If you want to play quiet music, light candles, wear a certain sweater or anything else to set the mood, that's great. Try to create a lasting ritual that will encourage you to return time and time again.

Finally, remind yourself that there is no real right or wrong way to meditate – simply find that place and space where you can clear your mind and connect with your breath, and that's all you need for a great year of meditation.

Week One: 1-7 Minutes of Meditation

If you expect to sit down and meditate serenely for 25 minutes on your first day, you're probably (honestly, definitely) setting yourself up for disappointment. So start small, simple and sweet – just one minute on day one. From there, you can add one minute each day this week. Of course, if one minute feels like a piece of cake, you're welcome to keep going, but without any pressure or expectation. This is a great way to build your base, and, if you want, you can go all the way up to the year you're meditating in: 13 minutes for 2013, 14 minutes for 2014 – use it as a way to celebrate where you are!

Try It: Set a timer for just one minute to start with. Sit comfortably, relax your shoulders and simply breathe in and out, noticing your breath as you let your thoughts go. It sounds so simple, but you just have to remind yourself to relax your thoughts, to come back to your breath, even if it's a million times. Try adding a minute a day throughout the week.

Tip of the Week: Experiment: with the time of day, the length of your meditation practice, your location, your position, your focus. What works for you on Monday may not make any sense by Friday, so give yourself room to move and breathe your way into a consistent meditation practice. And if you need to stick with just one or two minutes all week, that's fine – meet yourself where you are.

Week Two: Counting

In the trend of keeping it simple to keep it going, you will simply count your breath this week, one minute at a time. Again, you'll use a timer and determine how long you want to meditate, but this time, you will count the number of breaths that you take each minute. You might notice that the number decreases the longer you sit. It's a good reminder that the more you slow down and mono-task, instead of constantly multi-tasking, the more your breath, mind and body will slow down, too. This is also a good one for people with chatty minds – when you just focus one breath and one minute at a time, the time flies. When I do this meditation, I'm often taking about 15 breaths a minute when I start and can get down to as little as four after just a few minutes.

Try It: If you can set a timer/phone/watch to gently beep at one-minute intervals, that's ideal, otherwise, you can keep your eyes partially open to watch a second-hand. Start with five minutes of counting meditation and see if you can work up to 10 by the end of the week. Watch and count your breath.

Tip of the Week: Try this activity when you're stressed out, busy or a little frantic and notice how fast you're breathing. Then try it another day when you're feeling much calmer. It's interesting to notice how much your natural breath can vary based on your emotional state or schedule.

Week Three: Exhale

Feeling stressed or frazzled by life, to-dos or maybe even your new meditation practice? Then it's time to focus on exhaling. Exhales are more soothing and calming than inhales, and they might be just what the meditation doctor ordered this week. If you've ever taken a big, loud sigh out, you already recognize the magic of the exhale!

Try It: You can try this two ways: 1) Sit comfortably with your eyes closed, and simply notice your exhales. Let the inhales happen naturally and focus your attention on those lovely, soothing exhalations; 2) Breathe in for about three counts and breathe out for about six; if that feels good, extend it to four and eight, trying to make the exhale twice as long as the inhale, so you can really focus on releasing and letting go.

Tip of the Week: Whether you're seated or reclining, place your hands on your belly while you try this one. You can feel the belly rise as you inhale and really fall as you exhale, helping you to stay more focused on the sensations of the breath and truly enjoy that full exhale. It might also feel like an abdominal crunch without all the effort! And if you're alone, make some noise! Let yourself sigh out loud as you exhale to really get into the feel of letting go more.

Week Four: Inhale

If you're in the mood for a little energy this week, longer inhales can provide just that. Inhales can be more energizing, more lengthening and more encouraging than exhales, so this week you will experiment with longer breaths in, and notice how that feels.

Try It: Just like with exhalations, you can either: 1) Just notice your inhales. Feel the breath come in, notice your belly rise, experiencing your body opening up, and then let the exhales happen naturally; 2) Breathe in for about six counts and breathe out for about three; if that feels good, extend it to eight and four or even longer, trying to make the inhale twice as long as the exhale. Make sure the longer inhales don't feel like hyperventilation.

Tip of the Week: Again, don't be afraid to be heard – lightly constrict the back of your throat, and listen to the sound your breath makes as you inhale. Feel the vibration in the back of your throat and throughout your body. Counting to yourself as you breathe in and out can also help you stay more focused. Notice how you feel after a meditation practice focused on inhales, and if the answer is "more energetic," you can use this as a shot of natural caffeine anytime you need a quick boost.

Week Five: So Hum

So hum. So hum. So hum. (It's the meditators version of the Seven Dwarves' "hi ho, hi ho.") Say it out loud to yourself and listen to the natural flow of these two Sanskrit words which simply mean "I am." The goal is not to label anything after "I am" (for the next few minutes, you don't have to be a mom or a doctor or a sibling or a yogi, you just have to *be*), but rather to rest in these two syllables and the breath that carries them in and out.

Try It: You can either silently repeat these words to yourself or chant them aloud if that helps you stay more focused. Repeat "so hum" to yourself until it naturally reverberates, soaking up that lovely vibration. You can also try "so" as you inhale and "hum" as you exhale to create a steady rhythm.

Tip of the Week: You can also find recordings of so hum (in both song and chanting form), which can add a fun element to your meditation. Simply do an online search for "so hum" recording and you'll find a variety of voices that you can follow or sing along with!

Week Six: Lovingkindness

Whether it's Valentine's Day or you're just taking some time to appreciate yourself and the world around you, lovingkindness meditation is pretty lovely. This is one of my favorite meditations. You send good vibes to yourself, to someone you love, to someone you struggle with and to the world. It feels great!

Try It: After you find a comfortable seat, start with yourself and silently repeat these phrases (or others that resonate with you):

May I be safe.

May I be healthy.

May I be happy.

May I live with ease.

After a few rounds, envision someone you love or adore and silently send them those same loving thoughts:

May you be safe.

May you be healthy.

May you be happy.

May you live with ease.

Then, try the exact same thing, without any judgment or wrinkling of the face, with someone you struggle with. Finally, send those same messages of lovingkindness out to the world at large. Feel a warm glow from within.

Tip of the Week: Don't be afraid to picture someone you really, really struggle with for the third part of the meditation. It might feel fantastic to send them positive energy for a change, and it just might impact that challenging relationship.

Week Seven: Relax

If you find that meditating (or anything else in life – bills? traffic? relatives?) makes you a little tense, this meditation is the perfect antidote. It's all about relaxing and releasing from head to toe, softening everything in your body and your mind. I love to do this one in the evening as a way to totally unwind the day.

Try It: Lie on your back: Relax back, close your eyes and get comfortable. Then start at your feet and soften your toes, ankles, the tops and bottoms of your feet. If it takes a while, that's fine – there's no rush to relax. Slowly and mindfully make your way up from your feet to the crown of your head, relaxing and releasing every muscle, every bit of tightness or tension along the way. When you're finished, notice if there's anything that feels a little tight or stuck or achy and return to it with some soft exhales and some deep, relaxing breaths.

Tip of the Week: If your low back gets tight when you lie on your back, roll up a blanket or pillow under your knees and feel free to use a pillow under your head as well. This meditation is less about posture and more about pure relaxation.

Week Eight: Heart Chakra

As you breathe in and out during meditation, you might start to notice your heart beating in your chest. With that in mind, a meditation focused on the heart or "anahata" chakra can connect you to your center. Chakras are major energy centers along the spine, and the heart center is the fourth one, represented by the color green. When our heart chakra is open, we can give and receive love with ease, enjoy our relationships and generally feel in love with life, so this is definitely a meditation worth trying!

Try It: Sit comfortably and take a few deep breaths, feeling your heart beat. As you do so, imagine a bright, beautiful emerald green color around your heart center – green is the color of nature, life, nourishment. Feel the beauty and warmth here as you focus on breathing in positive, loving thoughts and exhaling anything you need to release around your heart. This is the center of the higher faculties of love, compassion, empathy and forgiveness. Breathe love in and out. Stay with this meditation anywhere from five to 20 minutes.

Tip of the Week: While we stay relatively still for a lot of meditations, if it feels good, you can circle your body in a clockwise direction as you focus on your heart center. You can also pay attention to your heart beating in your chest and sensations of love and warmth there.

Week Nine: Mantra

A mantra is any word or phrase that you can use to focus your mind, invite in something positive or create an intention for your day (or life). A few of the mantras I enjoy exploring during meditation include:

- Inhale, exhale
- Peace and calm
- My mind is clear, my body is strong, my heart is open.

(Your mantra might accidentally become, "why am I thinking so much today?" And that's normal, too.)

Try It: Take a moment to determine the best mantra for you, whether it's one word or syllable or a longer sentence or paragraph (just make it something that's easy to memorize, so you won't have to read it).

After finding a comfortable seat and your natural breath, focus all of your attention on your mantra. Whenever the mind wanders off, bring it compassionately back to your mantra. Stay this way for five to 20 minutes and rejoin the rest of your day, feeling refreshed, focused, enlivened.

Tip of the Week: If you find one word or phrase that works perfectly for you, great! Otherwise, feel free to try different options. You might prefer to keep it simple and simply breathe the word "peace" in and out. On the other hand, a longer sentence might help to keep your mind from wandering. If there's a day where you need a little energy, you can use "May I feel energized" as your mantra, and if there's a day where you need a little calm, you can use "As I breathe in, I feel calm. As I breathe out, I feel peace." You can make this really personal and effective.

Week Ten: Vacation Meditation

Who doesn't love vacation? A vacation meditation simply encourages you to focus on the beauty in your life, whether you're on holiday or are simply enjoying some relaxing time at home. It's about appreciating and noticing the sweet things in life. I try to remember to meditate when I'm traveling (it's really grounding if you're changing time zones and gives you the chance to slow down, smell the fresh air and enjoy where you are), but sometimes just breathing, enjoying some new sights and taking time to appreciate is all you need.

Try It: If you're literally on vacation, focus on the beauty of the sky, the different sights, sounds and smells, and your breath in a new place. If you're at home in your living room, close your eyes and imagine one of your favorite places. See yourself there – notice the sights, sounds, smells, tastes – everything surrounding you. Find a soft smile on your face and breathe that in and out.

Tip of the Week: If vacation meditation means "take a vacation from meditation" to you this week, give yourself permission to take a break, not worry about it and come right back. Be kind to yourself and remember that building a new habit takes time.

Week Eleven: Guided Meditation

Several times a year, the Chopra Center (as in Deepak Chopra, www.chopracenter.org) offers a free guided meditation based on a theme ("Who am I?", "mind-body health" and so on). This is a great chance to have someone else organize, prepare and deliver your daily meditation – all you have to do is show up! Meditations generally range from 10 to 20 minutes and can be downloaded for free during the 21 days (after that time, they sell the podcasts).

Try It: It's as simple as sitting back, relaxing and following along. Give yourself time and space, then simply press play and follow the instructions, which will generally center on your breath, your body, your thoughts. In addition to the Chopra Center, you can find other guided meditation podcasts online and through CDs.

Tip of the Week: If a lovely, soothing voice helps you get – and stay – in the mood, search for various online guided meditations, CDs or podcasts. There are a variety of free or inexpensive options available.

Week Twelve: Yoga Nidra

Following on the guided meditation theme, yoga nidra, also known as "yogic sleep," is like a conscious nap on your yoga mat. Each session can be a little bit different, but essentially, your yoga nap focuses on setting an intention, relaxing various parts of your body, visualization and other techniques designed to cultivate pure relaxation. In theory, you should feel as refreshed as if you'd just taken a nap (without falling asleep).

Try It: Google "yoga nidra" and look for a few free online podcasts, or ask someone to read a script for you. You might also be able to find local classes or workshops. This one does require the assistance of someone else's voice; if you're constantly opening your eyes to read the next stage in the script, you'll miss out on all the fun. All you have to do is follow along, relax and soak it up.

Tip of the Week: Try this one at night, right before you're planning on going to sleep, and see if it helps you drift off a little more easily, a little more peacefully. Last time we tried it at home, my husband fell asleep and started snoring, but a gentle nudge and giggle brought him back to the meditation.

Week Thirteen: Walking Meditation

It feels good to move, and walking meditation is great when you're feeling fidgety or simply having a hard time sitting. The concept is super simple – just walk and pay attention. Naturally, we breathe all day, every day, and we also walk (hopefully) quite a bit. Combining the two creates a mindful movement practice that is especially great for anyone who struggles to sit still or has back pain. And if you live in an area that has a labyrinth you can walk in, you can enjoy a maze, movement and breathing all in one! Lakes, rivers, bike paths and hiking trails are also great spots for walking meditation, but you can do this anywhere – on a loud and busy street, in your office building, even in your basement!

Try It: Take a walk with just yourself – no music, no company, no phone – just you and your body. It can be a long stroll around a lake or a lunchtime errand; it doesn't matter as long as you can pay attention. Feel your feet on the earth. If you can be barefoot, feel your toes spread out. Feel the air on the skin, the way your arms move. Keep a soft focused gaze and just notice your breath and your body moving.

Tip of the Week: If you want to really slow it down, try inhaling on one foot, exhaling on the other, or even further, inhale the heel of one foot and then exhale as you place the ball and toes of that same foot on the earth. Breathe.

Week Fourteen: Reading Meditation

If you're a bit of bookworm or are interested in learning even more about different types of meditation, different benefits and different schools of meditation, then this meditation is for you. It gives you another chance to take your meditation practice out into the world. This week is all about reading all about meditation (and trying to do so mindfully, rather than just rushing through the words).

Try It: The options are limitless – you can buy or check out a book or two on meditation, find articles in magazines, do online searches, whatever you prefer. I love anything by Sally Kempton, the *Elephant Journal*, the *Yoga Journal*, *Meditations on the Mat* by Rolf Gates and even articles in popular magazines that approach meditation from a really straightforward and simple perspective. The more you know, the more options you have.

Tip of the Week: Try to dedicate at least 10 minutes a day to reading about meditation, and then, if possible, dedicate another 10 minutes to trying out anything new that you've learned. Be adventurous in seeking out new sources and ideas.

Week Fifteen: Eating Meditation

Take a deep breath and a small bite – who wouldn't love eating or food meditation? This one is all about paying attention to what you eat, how you eat, how you taste and how you enjoy your food. Rather than racing through meals as so many of us tend to do, you will take the time to focus on the color, texture, taste and feel of every bite, which really helps you slow down (and, actually, eat a little less. There are diets based on this method that allow anything and everything, as long as you are super mindful about eating.).

Try It: Allow extra time for your meals this week and really focus in on your meal or snack. How did you prepare it? How does it look on your plate? How does it smell? What is its texture? What colors pop out? What are you most looking forward to? Then, rather than taking huge gulps, take small bites and truly taste your food. Enjoy your food. Make it a moving meditation of sorts.

Tip of the Week: If you have been thinking about a certain change in your diet (vegetarian, gluten-free, more fruits and veggies), this might be the perfect week to try it. You can really pay attention to how the new diet makes you feel and how your food tastes.

Week Sixteen: In and Out Meditation

Our days and lives are busy and hectic, but that doesn't mean we have to lose awareness and insight. When you use your day as your meditation practice, you will find many, many opportunities to pause, notice, breathe and simply take it all in. This week's focus allows you to zoom out and in throughout your day, noticing the big stuff, the little stuff and the in-between stuff.

Try It: Throughout your day, imagine a zoom lens look at your activities as well as a wide-angle view of your activities. As you zoom in, pay attention to the smallest details – how do your feet feel on the floor as you walk towards the kitchen for breakfast? What flavors of your morning smoothie really stand out? How does your hand feel when it wraps around the steering wheel? To zoom out, notice the space around you, the view, the sounds, the smells, the broader experience. Zoom in and out on everything you do throughout the day, from brushing your teeth, to having a meeting at work, to exercising, to meeting a friend for a cup of coffee.

Tip of the Week: Alternate back and forth between zooming in and out to notice both the small details and the larger experience of your day; notice how this moving, full-day meditation feels and affects your experience of the day as a whole.

Week Seventeen: Let Go

Let go of the things that weigh you down, let go of the things that hold you back, just let go – this is a great mantra and meditation practice any week of the year. This is also a simple healing meditation that feels good and focuses the mind. It's a nice one early in the morning as you let go of anything that might hold you back during your day and equally lovely at night as you release anything that's built up over the day. Sometimes my neck feels longer and my shoulders feel more relaxed after just a few minutes of this meditation.

Try It: Find a comfortable seated or reclined position and drop into your breath, focusing more on your inhales and exhales and less on your thoughts. When you're ready, introduce "let go" – "let" on the inhale and "go" on the exhale. Simply repeat these words silently to yourself for five to 20 minutes and then pause and notice the effect of these simple, powerful words.

Tip of the Week: If anything bubbles up that you need to let go of, simply let it go with your next exhalation and return to the "let go" breathing pattern, rather than getting all caught up in an emotion or a thought. Just let go.

Week Eighteen: Three-Part Breathing

Pranayama is also known as "breath control," but I like to think of it more as freedom of breath, rather than something so rigid. A particular type of breathwork, three-part breath helps you breathe deeply and expand your lung capacity. Another bonus? Focusing on your breath in a specific way gives your mind something to do and you'll feel amazing after.

Try It: Three-part breath is also known as complete breathing, and it's just that: breathing in three parts. Sit or lie back and start with the belly breath, feeling your belly expand and contract as you inhale and exhale deeply. Once that feels good, add on the second part: Breathe half of your air into the belly, then expand the second part of the breath up into the ribcage. Exhale from the top down, drawing the rib cage together, then the belly in toward the spine. Finally, breathe about one-third of your air into your belly, one-third to open up the rib cage and one-third to the top of the collarbones. It's a big, full breath in. Exhale the same way from top to bottom. Repeat several rounds, then allow breath to return to normal.

Tip of the Week: If this meditation makes you feel dizzy or light-heated, pause and breathe naturally for a few minutes. Otherwise, try to really lengthen the breath in and the breath out and send it into any tight spaces.

Week Nineteen: Frustration Meditation

To put it mildly, we all have frustrating weeks, which will make putting frustration meditation into action pretty easy. You can tune into a specific frustrating situation for this meditation and then let it go (as much as possible) in the same session, which feels pretty fantastic. (This week is also a good reminder that meditation, too, can be frustrating sometimes, but the fruits of it are well worth any tough days.)

Try It: Find a comfortable seated or reclined position and find your natural breath for a few moments. Then, allow yourself to think of something that's really been frustrating you – a person, an issue at work, an experience – and really feel that frustration in your body. Notice what it feels like to be frustrated – what tightens up, what constricts. Then focus on relaxing each part of your body, taking some deep exhales out of your mouth to try to release the frustration, anger or tension. Notice what that feels like in your body. Remind yourself that everything is temporary. Try to breathe in feelings of peace and calm and breathe out any lingering frustration.

Tip of the Week: When you get frustrated (whether you're meditating or not), remind yourself that this isn't the first time you've been frustrated, nor will it be the last. Likewise, panicking and freaking out never really help. A few moments of calm can help ease any frustration.

Week Twenty: Driving Meditation

If you always seem to be on the road again, driving meditation can help clear your mind and give you a new perspective at the wheel (or on the bus, train, taxi, you name it). It's simple – driving and breathing. The difference, of course, is paying attention to the breath, drawing it in and out deeply. It makes the ride more enjoyable, and releases some of the frustration you might feel at other drivers, construction, traffic or your to-do list. This is a great way to spend your time if you find yourself in rush-hour traffic, running late or on road trips, when you can unwind into the rhythm of your breath and the road.

Try It: Next time you get in your car, pause before you even turn the key. Notice your breath, the position of your body, the quality of your thoughts. Relax your shoulders and engage your core. Then slowly, turn the key and feel that vibration. As you drive, focus on taking long, slow deep breaths in and out, through your nose or your mouth. Let your breath create a moving meditation for you and your vehicle. Consider turning the radio down and just listening to your breath and the sounds of the open road.

Tip of the Week: Make sure you're still a safe driver when practicing driving meditation. Being present should make you more aware, but don't let the breath take you off into some other world while you're behind the wheel!

Week Twenty-One: Feeling Meditation

If you tend to bottle your feelings up or take them out on others in a not-so-healthy way, feeling meditation can help you deal with your emotions more productively and patiently. Sometimes we get so in tune with our heads that we stop listening to our hearts, so this is a perfect way to reconnect with what's going on inside.

Try It: To start, take a few deep, slow breaths as you bring your focus inside. Then ask yourself, "What am I feeling right here and right now?" After you detect any feelings, you can ask, "Is it pleasant or unpleasant?" and "Can I maintain these feelings or emotions or do I need something more or something else?" Just breathe into whatever sensations arise, acknowledging your feelings without identifying with them. This isn't a matter of right and wrong, but of noticing what's there. Use your exhales to let go of anything – judgment, doubt, expectation, jealousy, grief, anxiety – that is no longer serving you. Breathe in fresh air and fresh energy with every inhale and let go a little more with each exhale.

Tip of the Week: Sometimes the feelings that come up when we meditate are intense, and that's ok. If you find yourself crying, giggling, scowling or anything else, just notice what's coming up, give yourself the time to feel it, then settle back into your breath.

Week Twenty-Two: Chakra Meditation

The chakras, the major energy centers in the body that run along the spine, can provide the basis for many different meditations – you can focus on one at a time (like we did with the heart) or on each one in a series. It gives you a chance to focus on different areas in your body and your life where you need a boost, and it's pretty cool to boot.

Try It: The following chakra meditation can help you open up, notice and connect:

- Start with your focus at the base of your space, the root chakra, represented by the color red with a focus on survival, family, security and self-preservation. When this energy center is open, we feel rooted, grounded and confident that we can meet our core needs. When blocked, we may experience anxiety or worry. Take a deep breath and draw it down to the base of your spine, envisioning the color red and focusing on your connection to the earth. As you exhale, relax the muscles in your toes, feet and legs. Feel connected and grounded. Feel the density of your bones, the support structure of your body. Continue to breathe in and out, allowing your body to feel safe and secure.
- When you're ready, move up to the second chakra, just below the belly button. The color is orange and the focus is one-on-one relationships, desire, sensation and creativity. When this chakra is open, creative expressions occur naturally and we feel more connected to others. Keeping the root chakra open, take a deep breath in, and let the red energy heat up to a glowing orange. Relax your glutes, your belly, hips, and pelvis. Breathe warm orange energy into the second chakra. Feel the warm glow in your body. Tune

into any sense of warmth or vibration, and let it to grow, centering on this creative power within.

- Then, move up to your navel chakra at the solar plexus, envisioning a bright yellow, like sunshine. The focus is on personal power, strength, self-confidence. When open, you are capable of translating your intentions into reality. When blocked, you may feel frustrated or ineffectual. Take another fresh, deep breath in through your nose and as you exhale, let your attention settle in your middle, your center of gravity. As you meditate on this center of power and strength, breathe in bright yellow energy and continue to allow your stomach muscles to relax. The third chakra controls breathing and digestion, and your belly is the center of control and trust. It's all about your gut instincts. The energy from below continues to heat up. Feel the warmth from within.

- Next move to the heart center, the connection between the lower and higher chakras, which glows with an emerald green color and is our center of love and emotions. When open, we can give and receive love without fear or attachment and feel more connected. When blocked, we can feel isolated or alienated from others. Bring your focus to the center of your chest, centering your awareness on your heart and feeling it beat and grow stronger. The fourth chakra rules the heart and lungs and the color is green, nature's own color of life and nourishment. Here, you can find balance between yourself and the world. This is the also center of the higher faculties: love, compassion, empathy, forgiveness -- the center of pure unconditional love. Open your heart to others. Breathe love in and out.

- The next chakra is at the throat, represented by the color blue and the concepts of self-expression and creativity. When open and flowing, we can effortlessly express our authentic self, it helps us feel alive and empowered; when closed, we struggle to speak our truth. Relax and soften your tongue, vocal cords, neck muscles, shoulders, arms and hands. Let go of the word "should" that resides in "shoulders." Located here, the thyroid is a master regulator of other endocrine glands and the metabolism, hormone balances and immune function. Breathe in balance and equilibrium. Envision a cool blue light shining through your neck and throat, clearing out any constriction or discomfort. Let go of tension, relaxing from the jaw to the shoulders, and replace it with a feeling of open space. The throat center encircles your communication skills, artistic sense and capacity for innovation. Breathe into this creativity and capacity.

- The third-eye chakra resides in the space between the eyebrows and is represented by the color violet and your intuition and imagination. When open, we have a deep connection to our intuitive self, independent of the opinions of others, guided by our inner knowing. When blocked, there is a sense of self-doubt or distrust. Draw your awareness to the space between your eyebrows, exhaling to relax deeply and imagine that each breath has the effect of opening this third-eye center, like a window opening to a morning sunrise. Allow the brilliant light directly in, splashing a rainbow of color through your mind. This is the center of the quiet but powerful voice of intuition, where we can see beyond the ordinary limits of time and space. Feel connected to yourself and the world around you. Breathe in this beautiful violet energy.

- The seventh chakra, which is white or luminous, is at the crown of the head – our connection to the universe. When open, we feel more connected and aware, when closed, we are less aware of what's going on in the world around us and may feel heavy. Breathe into the crown chakra, which is like a thousand-petalled lotus opening up from the top of your head. Feel connected, wise, aware.

Finally, take a few deep breaths, blink your eyes open and feel your body and energy centers open as well.

Tip of the Week: If you come to one of these places and really feel something – maybe a lack of energy, maybe something vibrating – you can stay a little longer and really focus your time and attention there. You can also move up and down the spine pretty quickly and simply tune in to the energy at various places in your body at a given time.

Week Twenty-Three: Creativity out of the Box Meditation
Whether you're feeling creative this week or not, tapping into that wellspring of creativity inside that sometimes gets clouded over by to-do lists and general busyness can help you find that spark and celebrate it. We all have creativity, but we sometimes fail to look for it or to use it. This meditation can help you examine the contents of your mind and rediscover the power of your imagination, since we're all creative beings at heart.

Try It: You can either place an empty box in front of you or imagine an empty box there. Take a few moments to simply observe. Now, imagine that the box represents your mind: What do you see in the box? What might these things represent? Then, imagine removing each item one at a time from the box. What feelings or issues does this bring up? Without judgment, expectation or worry, simply notice what comes up. To close the meditation, imagine placing everything back in the box and closing the lid.

Tip of the Week: Another option for creativity meditation is to give yourself a few moments to focus on ways you can incorporate creativity into your work, your home or any part of your life, and breathe that focus in and out. Meditation makes me feel more creative, but I also signed up for a poetry class and a photography class as a way to fan those flames.

Week Twenty Four: Weight of the World Meditation

By adding a little weight to your legs, you can let go of a little weight off your shoulders and your mind. As someone or something (a weight) presses down firmly (but not painfully) on your quadriceps or thighs, the breath will start to deepen and expand automatically. This is one of those meditations that feels really, really good and can become addictive (in a good way).

Try It: If you have a great friend/partner/spouse/child who is willing to apply constant pressure to your thighs for 10-15 minutes, count yourself lucky! You can also use a weight, a sandbag, thick phone book or anything else that will provide even pressure to your thigh bones. Notice your breath for a few moments without the weight, and then notice how it deepens as you get more grounded and connected as you add weight to your legs. Focus on your breath and the sensations of being grounded as you breathe in and out.

Tip of the Week: Experiment with different amounts of weight – you can start lighter, around 10-15 pounds, and move up to as much as 30-40 pounds, depending on your frame and your preference.

Week Twenty Five: Do You Have an App for That? Meditation

Smart phones make everything, including meditation, a little more accessible. In particular, you can now use your iPhone or Android to research and download meditation apps with information on meditating as well as guidance – the number of mind-body apps continues to grow, so simply search for "meditation" or "breathing" and you'll find tons of options. If you love technology, this is a great way to integrate it with your meditation practice.

Try It: Using your smart phone, search for meditation-related apps to download. You can try one for a week or longer if you like. There are even apps that will beep at a certain time each day to remind you to stop, breathe and meditate. Feel free to experiment with different styles and opportunities.

Tip of the Week: If you're a budget-focused meditator, start with the wealth of free meditation app options before downloading anything that costs. And if you're more low-tech or no-tech, let your creativity shine and make up your own meditation this week!

Week Twenty Six: Divine Qualities Meditation

Some days and weeks we spend too much time with anger, irritation, frustration, impatience, confusion and doubt when we would benefit so much more from the divine qualities of love, compassion, gratitude, joy and peace. A meditation focused on exactly these qualities, then, is the perfect antidote for whatever ails you.

Try It: Get comfortable and find your breath. Starting with **love**, focus on your heart center and breathe love in and breathe love out. After a few minutes, transition to **gratitude**. You can focus on one person or experience or just soak up gratitude for a million different things. Then move on to **compassion** – imagine someone who is going through a major challenge and take a few moments to empathize with that person and send him or her positive energy. Next, take a few minutes to feel **joy** in your entire being as you breathe in and breathe out. Finally, soak up a few minutes of **peace and calm** as you feel all of these divine qualities in your mind, body and breath.

Tip of the Week: If there is one quality you could really use some more of in your life, then spend a few extra minutes with it. And as always, if there are other qualities or components that you'd like to invite it, by all means, make this practice personal.

Week Twenty Seven: Health Meditation

We have this one body, so it only makes sense to take care of it. Sometimes we might be great at this and sometimes we might neglect our health, so this week's meditation is designed to focus on feeling good and honing in on any aspect of your health that you'd like to improve or enhance. Whether you want to eat better, move more, stand taller, relax more or anything else, meditation is a healthy practice that can move you in the right direction.

Try It: Get comfortable and find your breath. Ask yourself, "How am I feeling right now?" "What, if anything, would I like to change or improve about my health?" "How can I go about doing just that?" Take a few minutes with your breath and these questions, and then breathe in the image of yourself doing the things you need to nurture yourself and take the best care of yourself. You might focus on one thing in particular or several healthy aspects in general.

Tip of the Week: Don't let this be an exercise in judgment. Try to focus on the positive, rather than tearing yourself down. This is an exercise in making healthy change. It's a great one to use if you've made a health-focused New Year's resolution that you'd like to return to, or if you could use some gentle reminders about making your health a priority.

Week Twenty Eight: Community Meditation

We're all connected, but we sometimes fail to recognize this powerful fact. When we realize how connected everyone and everything is, then we sometimes start to behave with others in mind, to live better and more intentionally. A community-focused meditation will help you recognize the community and support you have in your life.

Try It: After you find your comfortable seat and breath, take a few moments to just pause and notice. Then, start to examine the notion of community – what does it mean to you? Who comprises your community? How are you supported without even realizing it? How can you connect more with your community and give more? Breathe in this unconditional support, letting go of fear or doubt. Feel yourself surrounded by the energy and support of your community.

Tip of the Week: Let your definition of community be broad and fluid. It might be your community at work, at home, in your neighborhood, at your favorite coffee shop, in your yoga class or your faraway friends who keep close in touch.

Week Twenty Nine: Breath of Fire Meditation

Breath of fire meditation, which is also known as or "skull-shining breath" (it's not as scary as it might sound) is a warming, intense breath practice that will really activate your core (kind of like doing sit-ups with your breath). Start slow on this one and build up to more reps and more rounds.

Try It: Place your hands on your belly and focus on taking sharp, powerful exhales through your nose – let the inhales just happen naturally. Do one round of about 30 breaths. Pause, breathe deeply and try to repeat two more times. Then sit quietly and notice how your body feels.

Tip of the Week: If you're pregnant, overheated or tend to have anxiety, this meditation can be too heating, so simply skip it and return to one of your previous favorites.

Week Thirty: One Word Meditation

Sometimes, simplicity is best. One word. One idea. One quality. By focusing on one quality you could use a little more of in your life, you set yourself up for success and give yourself time to focus in on the things you most want and need. I love this meditation when I need to keep it simple and focused.

Try It: After you find yourself a comfortable space and a comfortable breath, ask yourself, "What one quality would I like to invite more of into my life this week?" Then breathe that word in and out, in and out, using it as your mantra for the day or the week.

Tip of the Week: If there are a variety of qualities you'd like to invite into your world this week, feel free to focus on a different one each day. Otherwise, if you'd like to really hone in on one thing, one quality, use that as your mantra for seven days in a row and see how you feel at week's end!

Week Thirty One: Cooling Meditation

When people get overheated, they tend to get a little cranky, frustrated, irritable and on edge, for good reason. The heat can really zap you. With that in mind, a cooling meditation can help defuse anger, soothe the body on a hot day and provide some perspective using both breath and imagery. (Likewise, this meditation can cool off a hot temper on any type of day.)

Try It: Sit comfortably and attempt to curl the sides of your tongue up into a u-shape (if you can't do it, no worries – it's a genetic thing. Instead, simply rest the tip of your tongue at the roof of your mouth). Inhale through your mouth, feeling the cool air at the back of the throat, and exhale through your nose. Take several deep, cool breaths this way and literally feel your body cool off. Alternately, when you simply focus on the word "cool," you can feel yourself cooling down and calming down a bit. Imagine cool air bathing your skin or cool water pouring on your head. Breathe this imagery and this word in and out and let off some steam.

Tip of the Week: If you're reading this in the middle of a cold snap, simply switch it around – take deep, warm breaths in and out through your nose only, feeling the body warm up from the inside out, and imagine heat, fire and warmth enveloping your body.

Week Thirty Two: Posture Meditation

By now, sitting up straight, relaxing your shoulders and grounding your sitting bones should be a little easier, so this week's meditation is all about posture, creating lift and space for your breath. If you tend to hunch forward, this meditation is a great reminder about the importance of posture.

Try It: Take extra time and care as you set up this week. Feel free to sit on a block, towel or blanket, making sure both sides of your body root down evenly. If your knees float up, place something under them so they are supported. Feel the uplift in your chest, back and crown of the head as your shoulders soften. Let your palms rest face up on your knees. Close your eyes and relax your face. As you inhale, imagine your spine getting longer as your breath moves up the front of the body. As you exhale, feel that release as your breath moves down the back of your body. Focus on your breath and the beautiful length in your amazing spine as you breathe in and out. Feel yourself getting taller as you breathe. Find the balance between effort and ease as you breathe length in and out.

Tip of the Week: While posture is important, so is being pain-free. If sitting in the middle of the room is miserable, then sit with your back against a wall, so you have support. If it helps, imagine bright light moving up and down your spine as you breathe.

Week Thirty Three: Tonglen Meditation

Tonglen meditation is a more advanced style of meditation which refers to "giving and taking." In this meditation, you take on the suffering of another person and in return, send out joy, happiness or comfort. You can use this heartfelt meditation to send out good wishes to someone in your life who could use some healing, happiness or good health.

Try It: Sit comfortably and imagine someone you know who is experiencing difficulty, whether it's a health issue, a troubled relationship, a protracted job search or something else. Then, breathe in your desire to take away that person's pain, fear or hurt. With your next breath out, send that person joy, bliss, health, happiness or whatever they need. You breathe in that person's pain so that they can find greater wellness, and breathe out whatever they need to find happiness. You can continue with one person or move to a more global desire to alleviate pain and suffering through breath and meditation.

Tip of the Week: Often, as you focus on someone else, you'll end up confronting your own pain or fear or jealousy or hurt, honoring the fact that many of us are in the same boat. You can do this practice for yourself as well and for the many others who are experiencing similar issues.

Week Thirty Four: Sky-gazing Meditation

If you live away from the city lights, there's nothing like a starry night, where you can just get mesmerized by the twinkling lights of stars and planets overhead. This meditation is inspired by the natural world and is great for a wandering mind, since it doesn't require a strict focus. And it works in the city, too – sometimes I focus on a cloud, the moon or anything else that's bright in the night sky.

Try It: Simply find an outdoor location that gives you a great view of the sky. Your eyes will stay open with a soft gaze that allows you to see the sky in broad strokes. You can even imagine that you have eyes in the back of your head, giving you an amazing 360-degree view of the world overhead. You don't have to look for anything in particular. Rather, just sit with the awareness of the natural beauty overhead, your breath, your thoughts, your being. Feel your connection to the earth below and above.

Tip of the Week: If taking in broad expanses of sky is a little distracting or overwhelming, simply close your eyes for a few moments until you feel focused again. If it's chilly out, bundle up so you're not distracted by chattering teeth. And even if you can't see many stars, just enjoy the beauty of sitting outside in the natural world.

Week Thirty Five: Forgiveness Meditation

Sometimes we think that forgiveness is more about the other person than ourselves, not pausing to realize that when we hang onto an old wound, hurt, slight or anger, we do more damage to ourselves than anyone else. While forgiveness is not always easy, it allows us to move forward and move on, so a week of forgiveness meditation can be really powerful and impactful.

Try It: You can either bring to mind an individual or a situation that could use a little forgiveness on your part or simply focus on the concept more generally. Take a few moments to really feel whatever hurt or anger is still inside of you and then try to relax that with a few exhales, breathing in love and breathing out healing. If it helps, you can silently say, "I forgive you" as you meditate.

Tip of the Week: Sometimes we think that some situations and people are simply unforgivable, but it helps to recognize that most people are doing the best they think they can with what they have at any given time. Combine compassion with your forgiveness meditation for extra oomph.

Week Thirty Six: Belly Breath

If you've recently had a chance to watch a baby breathe, then you know exactly what to do for this meditation (and we all do, we just forget sometimes). Belly breathing means really expanding the belly as you breathe in, and then letting it fall completely as you breathe out. It's simple and effective and calming.

Try It: This sweet and satisfying practice is all about focusing on the belly, and it's a little easier to do so when you're on your back. As you relax down onto your back, let your belly be soft. As you breathe in, feel it expand, then breathe out, drawing the belly back toward the spine. Feel the fullness in the center of your body. Continue to take deep and full breaths, focusing on the movement in your abdomen. Stay and breathe for as long as you like.

Tip of the Week: You can place your hands on your belly and really feel it rise and then drop to help you visualize and get in touch with this meditation even more. Envision a happy baby and smile to yourself.

Week Thirty Seven: Change Meditation

Everything is always changing, and that includes ourselves. You're not quite the same person you were when you woke up this morning. Sometimes these changes are welcome, and others times, not so much. But, since change is inevitable, learning to meet it with an attitude of openness will serve you much better than a body of resistance.

Try It: Take a few moments to contemplate a change in your life – whether it's something you'd like to make (eat more fruits and veggies) or something that's already happening (a relationship ending). Notice what sensations and emotions come up when you focus on this change. See where you can soften and release a little tension. Could you "change" your reaction to change to prompt a brighter outcome? Then, sit and breathe the word "allow" in and out as you focus on creating more room for change in your life.

Tip of the Week: Don't be afraid to contemplate a very big or a very scary change in this meditation; sometimes meeting change with patience and kindness can allow some of the terror or panic to soften a little. You can also breathe a little deeper, to fill your body up with energy, and to let go of resistance.

Week Thirty Eight: Question and Answer Meditation

As you may have realized, when you get quiet and clear and calm, it's not unusual to have powerful insights. Sometimes, it's simply "My stomach is growing and I'm really hungry," but sometimes, you can find answers to the major questions in your life. This week's meditation is about formulating a question and then being still enough to allow the answer to bubble up.

Try It: Whether you have one question you want to focus on all week or seven different questions, take the time to formulate your question before you sit down to meditate, and then set an intention to receive some insight. This could be anything from, "What do I really want out of my career?" to "How can I enhance my relationship with my mom?" to "What's next?" As you breathe in the question, see if anything comes up. Feel free to keep a notepad nearby if you'd like to write down any answers. Don't get frustrated if this takes some time, just practice being quiet and listening to any inner words of wisdom.

Tip of the Week: If any emotions arise, let them. Notice, breathe and relax into the sensation. Whether you follow the answers that come immediately or over time, meditation can help you find answers to both serious and light-hearted questions, give your relationships a boost and offer some much-appreciated clarity.

Week Thirty Nine: Five Senses Meditation

We certainly use our eyes a lot, but don't always take in as much information as we could with our other senses. A sensory meditation encourages the use of all five senses to focus in on the present moment and the beauty of your sight, sound, smell, touch and taste.

Try It: Keep your eyes slightly open to start and notice what you can see: What colors, shapes, items and shadows do your eyes take in? Can you still see them when your eyes close? And what do you see with your eyes shut? Next move on to smell: What smells – subtle or profound – can you distinguish? What are your favorite smells? Then, listen carefully: What do you hear with your eyes shut? Your own breath? The wind? Other people moving around? Just take the sounds in without attaching to or judging anything. Then, shift to touch: How do your hands feel as they rest on your legs? How is your body connected to the earth? Can you feel the air on your skin? Get sensitive to the slightest sensation of touch. Finally, focus on taste: Whether it's the lingering taste of an apple, the flavor of a piece of a gum or the imagined taste of your favorite food, let your mouth water.

Tip of the Week: This is another meditation that you can do anytime and anywhere. As you move through your day, notice sounds more. Pay attention to how your clothes feel on your skin. How a fresh tomato tastes. How the sky looks in the morning and at night. How your morning coffee smells.

Week Forty: Music Meditation

While most meditation music trends towards the mellow, this week you have the opportunity to experiment with *any* kind of music you want. If you can get in touch with your breath while listening to Metallica or Garth Brooks, that's perfect. Music is very powerful, so select your tunes with care.

Try It: Set yourself up for meditation in a seated or reclined position and play some tunes – something you love, something you've never heard, it's entirely up to you. You can experiment with different music genres throughout the week. Then notice your breathe along with the beat – do you breathe faster when the music speeds up? Does your breath slow down when you hear a melody you love? Do you tend to hold your breath during certain songs? Notice your breath and then try to expand it into the music.

Tip of the Week: While you can try any piece of music you fancy, be mindful of the words – if a song has negative language, that can seep into your thoughts and influence your meditation. And if you need to sing along, sing out – you have to breathe to sing, so that, too, can be a form of meditation.

Week Forty One: Alternate Nostril Breathing

Another type of specific breathwork, alternate nostril breathing is said to balance the hemispheres of the brain and the entire body, while focusing your mind (and clearing your sinuses – you might want some tissues nearby when you practice this one).

Try It: Sit up straight and place your left hand face up on your knee; connect your thumb and first finger. With your right hand, bend your first and middle finger in toward your palm. Exhale completely, then use your thumb to close the right nostril. Inhale through the left side, then close the left nostril with your ring finger. Exhale through the right side. Inhale right, pause, close, exhale left. That's one round. Repeat, repeat, repeat.

Tip of the Week: You can also experiment with holding the breath at the top: Breathe in through the right nostril for four counts, hold for four, breathe out left for four, hold for four, and so on. Experiment with the length of the breath and see if you can expand it to six, eight or even 10 counts. If it bothers your fingers to tuck them in toward your palm, you can also rest them above the bridge of your nose.

Week Forty Two: Nature-Inspired Meditation

This week's meditation is based on a meditation from Buddhist monk, scholar and writer Thich Nhat Hanh and provides some beautiful imagery as a focal point. I love to practice this one outside, whether on my front porch, near the lake or on a walk.

Try It: Take a moment to get comfortable, then repeat the following phrases to yourself, focusing on each one for one to five minutes:

Breathing in, I see myself as a flower.

Breathing out, I feel fresh.

Breathing in, I see myself as a mountain.

Breathing out, I feel solid.

Breathing in, I see myself as still water.

Breathing out, I reflect things as they truly are.

Breathing in, I see myself as space.

Breathing out, I feel free.

Tip of the Week: If there are other natural images that would inspire you (the sky, trees, a meadow), you can add those to the meditation as well. Really feel the qualities of freshness, solidity, reflection and freedom as you move through this lovely meditation.

Week Forty Three: Empty Coat Sleeves

This moving meditation is a lot of fun, but you might want to find a private place to try it out, so that you can really get into the motion (or do it with a friend and have some fun swaying around together). It evokes the idea of wearing a coat with empty sleeves that effortlessly sway from side to side as your body moves.

Try It: Stand up with your feet a little wider than hip-width distance apart and knees slightly bent. Let your arms hang loose, then gently sway your arms and torso from side to side. Inhale every time you come through center, exhale every time you twist to one side. Increase speed slowly, then eventually slow it back down. Stand in stillness for another minute or two to pause and absorb.

Tip of the Week: You can breathe in through your nose and out through your mouth for this one if that helps you breathe a little deeper. Really get into the movement and motion and let your body feel free and easy.

Week Forty Four: Breath Retention

Breath retention meditation gives you a chance to hold your breath in, further develop your lung capacity and simply pause in the middle of things. When you go to hold the breath, you can tuck your chin to your chest, and when you're ready to release, you'll lift your chin up to parallel again.

Try It: Simply inhale for about four counts, pause as you tuck your chin to your chest, hold for about four counts, and then lift your chin and exhale for four counts. You can play around with the counts and even increase the retention to a longer rate than the inhale and exhale.

Tip of the Week: Do not perform this one if you are pregnant, have high blood pressure, glaucoma or any other reason that you shouldn't hold your breath. You can start slow and build up to longer holds.

Week Forty Five: Opposites Meditation

We have to learn to live with the good days and the bad, the sorrow and the sweetness, the victories and losses. While we might like it if every day was sunny, fun and filled with pleasure, the challenging circumstances help us appreciate the bright days that much more. A meditation of opposites helps you breathe in qualities that you'd like more of in your life, and then breathe out their opposite, so no matter what is going on in the rest of your life, you feel grounded in the center.

Try It: You can use the following ideas to start, and then proceed on with your own (or focus on one or two items in the list that really resonate with you this week).

- Inhale joy, exhale sorrow.
- Inhale peace, exhale chaos.
- Inhale moderation, exhale excess.
- Inhale focus, exhale distraction.
- Inhale health, exhale illness.
- Inhale humility, exhale ego.
- Inhale bravery, exhale fear.
- Inhale heart, exhale head.

Tip of the Week: Feel free to be creative here as you focus on breathing in the qualities you could use a little more of right now.

Week Forty Six: Family Meditation

Whether you adore every single member of your family and get together regularly or have a challenging relationship when it comes to your relatives, everyone can benefit from a family-focused meditation. This gives you the chance to reflect on your relationships, with gratitude for the good ones and insight for the not-as-easy ones, and determine if there are places you can relax into better family reunions and connections. What a perfect pre-holiday meditation!

Try It: After you get comfortable, envision your family as a whole – immediate and extended. See them as a circle. Try to breathe warm, positive energy into that image. Now, if there are any members in the circle who are really sticking out, focus on them individually. Why do you love this person? Why does that person drive you crazy? How can your reactions improve when it comes to these relationships? You might not get the answers you seek in one session or one week – be patient and give yourself time to mend or strengthen these major bonds. Close the meditation by sending out positive energy for your family circle.

Tip of the Week: If you have a particularly toxic relationship with one or two relatives in particular, determine how you can forgive, let go or release any hold that has on you. Breathe forgiveness in, let go as you breathe out.

Week Forty Seven: Still Lake of the Mind Meditation

Sometimes are minds are clear and calm, like a beautiful lake, while others they are more like the ocean, wavy, roiling, loud. This meditation is designed to evoke the former state as you imagine your mind as a pellucid lake that allows your thoughts to reflect back. I grew up at my grandparent's lake in Iowa and love to imagine that sweet spot during this sweet meditation.

Try It: Relax you mind and your shoulders. Begin to picture your mind as a still lake, calm, clear and placid. See what's reflected in the lake, and let any thoughts that arise just move like ripples that return to stillness. Breathe in this image and stillness for a few minutes, letting any thoughts go as the ripples become more still. Enjoy the beauty of the quiet lake. Then, picture a full moon rising in the back of your mind and see its bright reflection in the lake. Notice the light of the moon on the still lake; any thoughts are simply ripples that move into stillness. Take several breaths as you focus on this beautiful imagery. Finally, imagine the light of the moon shining from the back of your mind to the space between your eyebrows, and throughout your entire body, creating a warm. Breathe in this imagery and this warmth before slowly opening your eyes.

Tip of the Week: This is a great meditation to do at the lake, on the beach or near another body of water. Surround yourself with the very nature you're bringing to mind in your meditation.

Week Forty Eight: Vipassana Meditation

In a traditional, stripped-down Vipassana meditation, you notice your thoughts without focusing on them or judging them or expecting anything from them. (If you've read or watched "Eat, Pray, Love," you've had the pleasure of seeing the lovely Elizabeth Gilbert struggle with this very form of meditation.) This very pure form of meditation focuses on the breath and nothing more. It's both that simple and that complex. The word "Vipassana" means "to see things as they actually are."

Try It: The instructions for Vipassana meditation are short and sweet: Observe your breath. You simply observe what comes and what goes with the aim of cultivating focus and calm. Naturally, your mind will wander, but do your best to simply bring it back to your next breath.

Tip of the Week: This traditional, ancient form of meditation is said to lead to ultimate enlightenment, so if it seems difficult at first, don't give up (rather, "enlighten" up!).

Week Forty Nine: Healing Meditation

Whether you are feeling a little beat up or run down, or have someone in your life who could use a little healing and comfort, the following meditation can help you focus on nurturing, health and wholeness. Healing can be physical, emotional, mental – you name it.

Try It: Envision a circle – the universal symbol of wholeness – that is divided into four quarters. Imagine that each of these four quarters is a window that you can look through. Look through each of the windows to create a picture or vision – it can be anything that springs to mind, something that you would like to lay your eyes on. Just pause and see it clearly. Now, imagine that the circle is radiating out a bright healing light which can fill your mind and your body with soothing, healing energy and warmth. Feel and envision that warm glow. Soak it up. When you feel warmer, lighter, healthier, you can let the image fade and return to your breath.

Tip of the Week: This is a meditation that you can do alone or with a group focused on health and healing. You can also envision that warm, bright light traveling up and down your spine.

Week Fifty: Just Be Meditation

We spend a lot of time criticizing ourselves, judging ourselves and altogether not appreciating ourselves. Whether it's our weight, our job, our relationships, our to-do list, our family or something else, many people find it easier to see the bad than the good, to notice the dark over the light. So this meditation is all about appreciating yourself *exactly as you are* – right here, right now.

Try It: Take a few deep breaths in through your nose, and then out through your mouth. As you exhale, feel your shoulders drop and notice your body and mind letting go a little. When you feel settled, silently repeat the following to yourself: I am perfect just as I am. I have enough. I am enough. These statements can remind you of your inherent worth and give you a chance to pause and truly appreciate exactly who you are.

Tip of the Week: If the "should," "would" or "could" comes up, let the thought go with your next exhale. This meditation isn't about improving or changing or challenging, it's all about being at peace with exactly who you are, where you are, what you are in the moment.

Week Fifty One: Life as Meditation

Life is a pretty good teacher, whether we are ready for the lesson or not. We learn discipline, patience, triumph, understanding and so much more simply by virtue of living each day as it comes. This week's meditation takes advantage of that fertile ground and uses your life as the actual meditation.

Try It: When you wake up tomorrow, pay attention. How does it feel to stretch? To stand up? To eat breakfast? How much attention can you pay to everything you do – whether it's a habit or a rarity – throughout your days? Let your meditation practice center on your day-to-day activities this week, giving extra time and attention to how you move through the world, how you breathe as you move and how it feels to be uniquely you. Where can you breathe a little easier? Where can you let go? What life lessons are surfacing this week?

Tip of the Week: Let your entire week be a meditation practice. Whether you are cooking dinner, walking to the bus, watching a movie, hanging out with a friend or preparing for bed, be as mindful as possible about every single thing you do. Then notice how that feels. Truly, our entire life can be a moving meditation when we learn to pay attention, slow down and breathe deeply.

Week Fifty Two: Gratitude Meditation

We're pretty good about practicing gratitude and gratefulness on Thanksgiving, but don't often give it much thought the rest of the year. When you're grateful, you're more aware of the good things in your life and less likely to get sidetracked by the not-as-good. Gratitude can fill your heart up and make the world a more beautiful place.

Try It: Silently ask yourself, "What am I grateful for right now?" You might prefer to focus on one person, place or experience, or a whole slide show of images might pass through your mind. Simply take it all in as you breathe in and out, appreciating all of the little and small bits of goodness in your life. Notice how amazing gratitude feels. Before you open your eyes, soak in the sensations of gratitude.

Tip of the Week: This is one of those meditations you can practice every single day and really benefit from. When you're stuck in traffic, ask yourself what you're grateful for. When your baby is crying, ask yourself what you're grateful for. When you have 30 hours of work and 3 hours to do it in, ask yourself what you're grateful for. You can remind yourself of gratitude anytime and anywhere. You might just realize how much you have to be grateful for.

Week 53 and Beyond

Congratulations on completing your year of meditation!

When I dedicated myself to a year of meditation, I did not meditate every single day and I was not perfect, but I did breathe deeper, find some meditations that I absolutely loved and even started teaching a meditation class. I've come to love meditation *almost* as much as I adore yoga, and appreciate the fact that I can do it anytime, anywhere.

I hope you feel calmer, happier, more grounded, more aware, more yourself. Your meditation journey can continue by repeating any or all of the 52 meditations on a regular basis. If there are one or two meditations that really work for you, stick with them or feel free to make up your own – consistency is the key to getting all the benefits and beauty out of your meditation practice.

Be curious and open. Search for free meditations online, look up a few ideas in a book, find a meditation group or meditate with a friend.

Just keep breathing.

Inhale, exhale, inhale, exhale…

www.ingramcontent.com/pod-product-compliance
Lightning Source LLC
Chambersburg PA
CBHW060003300526
45794CB00003B/1067